CORTISOL-YOUR BODY HORMONE:

Monitoring Cortisol

Tips on the best way to upgrade your physical condition, weight, fertility, and pressure management.

By

Kay J. Johnson

Copyright ©

All right reserved no piece of this book might be delivered in entire or to a limited extent without approval from the distributor, extracted regarding a survey in an electronic distribution, paper, and magazine, nor may any of this book be reproduced, stored in a recovery framework or sent in any structure without approval from the distributor.

Legal Disclaimer

This book is composed to proffer sound data and supportive tips, including the sentiments and exploration of the writer concerning some essentially clinical data.

This book isn't planned to replace the exhortation of a clinical practitioner, also this book is not to be taken to replace rule proposals or advance explicit treatments for individual cases. A proper discussion is required concerning your well-being before embracing any ideas in this book. The writer and distributor explicitly repudiate any liability, loss, or risk, that is caused by utilizing this book.

Table of content

Introduction

The major duty of each hormones is to send messages to various parts of the body. The messages they send and where they send them rely upon which sort of chemical we are discussing. Insulin, for example, keeps track of your glucose, while melatonin lets your body know when now is the ideal time to nod off. Most chemicals are made inside little organs called organs, and the principal occupation of these organs is typically to deliver explicit chemicals into the circulatory system so they can take their messages where they should go. Cortisol is made in your two adrenal organs — there's one in every kidney. The adrenal organs know when to make and deliver cortisol given a kind of continuous discussion between two distinct pieces of the cerebrum: the pituitary organ and the nerve center. Together, the adrenal organs, the pituitary organ, and the nerve center are known as the HPA pivot.

The cortisol level in your body normally vacillates throughout the day in a cadence set by the mind. "There are times in the day when cortisol is exceptionally low and times when it goes up very high.

It begins to go up somewhere in the range of two and three AM and has a pinnacle somewhere close to eight and nine AM, and afterward steadily declines during the day (with a couple of little increments) until around four or five PM, when the levels are exceptionally low and remain as such up until two a.m. returns around. There are trillions of cells in your body, and a larger part of them have receptors for cortisol, implying that cortisol can tie to practically any cell and change its capabilities. For this reason, cortisol is so significant — it assumes a part in basically every framework in the body.

Chapter One

What is Cortisol?

Cortisol

Cortisol is a steroid chemical that your adrenal, the endocrine organs on top of your kidneys, produce and deliver. Cortisol influences a few parts of your body and primarily controls your body's reaction to stretch.

What is cortisol?

Cortisol is a glucocorticoid chemical that your adrenal organs produce and deliver.

Chemicals will be synthetic substances that coordinate various capabilities in your body by bringing messages through your blood to your organs, skin, muscles, and different tissues.

These symptoms guide your body and know when to do it.

Glucocorticoids are a kind of steroid chemical. They smother aggravation in your substantial tissues as a whole and control digestion in your muscles, fat, liver, and bones. Glucocorticoids additionally influence rest wake cycles.

Your adrenal organs, otherwise called suprarenal organs, are little, triangle-formed organs that are situated on top of every one of your two kidneys. They're a piece of your endocrine framework.

Cortisol is an essential hormone that influences pretty much every organ and tissue in your body. It assumes numerous significant parts, including:

- Directing your body's pressure reaction.
- Helping control your body's utilization of fats, proteins, and carbs, or your digestion.
- Smothering irritation. Directing circulatory strain.
- Directing glucose.

- Helping control your rest wake cycle.

Your body ceaselessly screens your cortisol levels to keep up with consistent levels (homeostasis). Higher-than-typical or lower-than-typical cortisol levels can be unsafe for your well-being.

Cortisol is delivered every day to assist with managing your rest wake cycle, your digestion, and your invulnerable reaction from there, the sky's the limit. Each day, around 30 minutes after you are awake, your cortisol levels top to help

you prepare for the afternoon. Then they decline, arriving at their absolute bottom around midnight.

Organ Frameworks Included

Glucocorticoid receptors are available in practically all tissues in the body. In this manner, cortisol can influence almost every organ framework

- Nervous
- Immune

- Cardiovascular
- Respiratory
- Conceptive
- Outer muscle
- Integumentary

The arrival of cortisol is taken care of by the nerve center pituitary-adrenal (HPA) pivot. Corticotropin-delivering chemical (CRH) is delivered by the core (PVN) of the hypothalamus. It then follows up on the foremost pituitary to deliver adrenocorticotropic chemical (ACTH), which hence follows up on the adrenal cortex. In a negative criticism circle, adequate cortisol restrains the arrival of both ACTH and CRH. The HPA hub follows a circadian musicality. In this manner, cortisol levels will be high in the first part of the day and low around evening time.

Chapter Two

How Does Cortisol Function?

Your nerve center and pituitary organ - - both situated in your mind - - can detect, assuming your blood contains the right degree of cortisol. Assuming the level is too low, your cerebrum changes how many chemicals it makes. Your adrenal organs get on these signs. Then, they adjust how much cortisol they discharge.

Cortisol receptors - - which are numerous in cells in your body - - get and involve the chemical in various ways. Your requirements will vary from one day to another. For example, when your body is on guard, cortisol can modify or close down works that disrupt the general flow. These could incorporate your stomach-related or conceptive frameworks, your insusceptible framework, or even your development processes.
Once in a while, your cortisol levels can escape whack

After the stress or risks have passed, your cortisol level ought to quiet down. Your heart, pulse, and other body frameworks will fully recover.

Yet, imagine a scenario where you're under constant pressure and the caution button stays on.

It can wreck your body's most significant capabilities. It can similarly initiate various medical issues, including:

- Tension and melancholy
- Migraines
- Coronary illness
- Memory and fixation issues
- Issues with absorption
- Inconvenience resting
- Weight gain
- An excess of Cortisol

A knob (mass) in your adrenal organ or a growth in the cerebrum's pituitary organ can set off your body to make an excess of cortisol.This can result in a condition called Cushing disorder. It can prompt quick weight gain, skin that wounds effectively, muscle shortcomings, diabetes, and numerous other medical issues.

Too Little Cortisol

On the off chance that your body doesn't make enough of this chemical, you have condition specialists called Addison's illness. Generally, the side effects show up over the long haul. They include:

- Changes in your skin, such as dark scars and in skin folds.
- Being worn out constantly
- Muscle shortcoming that deteriorates
- Looseness of the bowels, queasiness, and regurgitating
- Loss of craving and weight
- Low circulatory strain
- On the off chance that your body isn't making sufficient cortisol, your primary care physician might recommend

dexamethasone, hydrocortisone, or prednisone tablets.

How does my body control cortisol levels?

Your body has an intricate framework to direct your cortisol levels.

Your nerve center, a little region of your mind engaged with hormonal guidelines, and your pituitary organ, a minuscule organ situated underneath your cerebrum, directs the creation of cortisol in your adrenal organs. At the point when the degrees of cortisol in your blood fall, your nerve center delivers corticotropin-delivering chemicals (CRH), which guides your pituitary organ to create adrenocorticotropic chemicals (ACTH). ACTH then, at that point, invigorates your adrenal organs to deliver and deliver cortisol.

To have ideal degrees of cortisol in your body, your nerve center, pituitary organ, and adrenal organs should be in every way working appropriately.

What tests can check cortisol levels?

Medical care suppliers can quantify your cortisol levels through blood, pee (pee), or salivation (spit) tests. They will figure out which test is best relying on your side effects.

What are typical cortisol levels?

The degree of cortisol in your blood, pee, and spit regularly peaks in the early morning and declines for the day, arriving at its most minimal level around noon. This example can change if you work a night shift and rest at various times.

For most tests that action cortisol levels in your blood, the ordinary reaches are:

6 a.m. to 8 a.m.: 10 to 20 micrograms for every deciliter (mcg/dL).
Around 4 p.m.: 3 to 10 mcg/dL.

Typical reaches can differ from one lab to another, from one opportunity to time, and from one individual to the next. If you want to get a cortisol level test, your medical care supplier will decipher your outcomes and let you know whether you want to get further testing.

What causes elevated degrees of cortisol?

Encountering unusually elevated degrees of cortisol (hypercortisolism) for a lengthy time frame is typically viewed as Cushing's disorder, which is an interesting condition. Reasons for higher-than-typical cortisol levels and Cushing's disorder include:

Taking a lot of corticosteroid prescriptions, like prednisone, prednisolone, or dexamethasone, for treatment of different circumstances.
Growths that produce adrenocorticotropic chemicals (ACTH). These are generally tracked down in your pituitary organ. All the more seldom, neuroendocrine growths in different

pieces of your body, for example, your lungs can cause high cortisol levels.

Adrenal organ cancers or inordinate development of adrenal tissue (hyperplasia), cause an overabundance creation of cortisol.

What are the complications of high cortisol levels?

The side effects of Cushing's condition rely on how raised your cortisol levels are.

Normal signs and side effects of higher-than-typical cortisol levels include:

Weight gain, particularly in front of you and midsection.

Greasy stores between your shoulder bones.

Wide, purple stretch blemishes on your midsection (stomach).

Muscle shortcomings in your upper arms and thighs.

High glucose, which frequently transforms into Type 2 diabetes.

Hypertension (hypertension).

Extreme hair development (hirsutism) in individuals allowed females upon entering the world.

Feeble bones (osteoporosis) and cracks.

What causes low degrees of cortisol?

Having lower-than-typical cortisol levels (hypocortisolism) is viewed as adrenal inadequacy.

There are two kinds of adrenal inadequacy: essential and auxiliary. The reasons for adrenal deficiency include:

Essential adrenal deficiency: Essential adrenal inadequacy is most generally brought about by an immune system response in which your resistant framework assaults sound cells in your adrenal organs for no great explanation. This is called Addison's illness. Your adrenal organs can likewise become harmed from a contamination or blood misfortune to the tissues (adrenal drain). These circumstances limit cortisol creation.

Optional adrenal deficiency: If you have an underactive pituitary organ (hypopituitarism) or pituitary growth, it can restrict ACTH creation. ACTH flags your adrenal organs to make cortisol, so restricted ACTH brings about restricted cortisol creation.

You can likewise have lower-than-ordinary cortisol levels in the wake of halting treatment with corticosteroid prescriptions, particularly if you quit taking them rapidly after an extensive stretch of purpose.

What are the symptoms of low cortisol levels?

Symptoms of lower-than-typical cortisol levels, or adrenal deficiency, include:

- Weakness.
- Inadvertent weight reduction.
- Unfortunate craving.
- Low circulatory strain (hypotension).

How can I reduce my cortisol levels?

Assuming you have Cushing's condition (extremely elevated degrees of cortisol) you'll require clinical treatment to bring down your cortisol levels. Treatment for the most part includes drugs and additional medical procedures. You'll likewise require clinical treatment assuming you have lower-than-ordinary cortisol levels.

As a general rule, however, there are a few ordinary things you can do to attempt to bring down your cortisol levels and keep them at ideal reaches, including:

- **Get quality rest:** Persistent rest issues, for example, obstructive rest apnea, sleep deprivation, or working a night shift, are related to higher cortisol levels.
- **Work-out consistently:** A few investigations have shown that normal activity further develops rest quality and decreases pressure, which can assist with

bringing down cortisol levels after some time.

- **Figure out how to restrict pressure and upsetting reasoning examples:** Monitoring your reasoning example, breathing, pulse and different indications of strain assists you with perceiving pressure when it starts and can assist you with keeping it from turning out to be more regrettable.

- **Practice profound breathing activities:** Controlled breathing animates your parasympathetic sensory system, your "rest and overview" framework, which helps lower cortisol levels.

- **Have fun and giggle:** Chuckling advances the arrival of endorphins and stifles cortisol. Taking part in leisure activities and fun exercises can likewise advance sensations of prosperity, which might bring down your cortisol levels.

- **Keep up with sound connections:** Connections are a significant part of our lives. Having tense and unfortunate associations with friends and family or collaborators can cause successive pressure and raise your cortisol levels.

When would it be a good idea for me to see my primary care physician about
my cortisol levels?

If you experience side effects of Cushing's condition or adrenal deficiency, contact your medical care supplier.

Cortisol is a fundamental chemical that influences a few parts of your body. While there are a few things you can do to attempt to restrict your pressure, and hence deal with your cortisol levels, some of the time having unusually high or low degrees of cortisol is beyond your control.

In the event that you experience side effects of high or low cortisol levels, for example, weight gain or misfortune and high or low circulatory strain, separately, reaching your medical services provider is significant. They can run a few straightforward tests to check whether your adrenal organs or pituitary organs are liable for your symptoms.

Chapter Three

The risks of burnout and what cortisol means for emotional wellness.

The Risks of Burnout.

To start with, it should be said: There's no disgrace in being worried about burnout. stress is named "the well-being pestilence of the 21st century. It's all over the place. And keeping in mind that burnout is frequently connected with the "making a difference" callings (like specialists or medical caretakers) or nurturing, it can influence anybody battling with ongoing pressure.

Shockingly, specialists don't settle on what causes burnout. Or on the other hand, even the way that they ought to characterize it. In any case, for the most part, burnout is acknowledged as a type of mental, profound, and actual depletion.

Burnout is a persistent pressure that has not been effectively made due. The three principal side effects are:

1. Sensations of energy consumption or depletion. That could include:

- Sleep deprivation.

- Ongoing weakness.

- Expanded diseases, like colds.

2. Expanded mental separation from one's job or feeling pessimistic toward it. That could include:

Despondency or general sensations of sadness.

Expanded uneasiness, skepticism, or outrage.

Lack of concern or separation.

3. Diminished viability. That could include:

Diminished inspiration and efficiency.

Inconvenience centering.

Feeling of disappointment and self-question.

Many side effects fall into these classifications, and it changes from one individual to another. So what's going on in our bodies that is causing this?

The Hormone Behind Persistent Pressure.

Eventually, burnout is a serious type of persistent pressure. That is significant because constant pressure prompts a key chemical, cortisol, to flood your body. Furthermore, that assumes a basic part in your well-being. Cortisol controls fundamental capabilities, like rest, assimilation, and, your invulnerable framework.

As a feature of your body's fight-or-battle or-freeze reaction, it likewise keeps you ready and prepared to confront dangers. That is the reason we produce more when focused.

Cortisol likewise manages your rest wake cycle, awakening you when levels normally increment each day and permitting you to fall (and stay unconscious) when levels drop around evening time. This is where we track down an association with burnout side effects. It's just plain obvious when ongoing pressure raises your cortisol levels, your rest is seriously jeopardized. Abruptly, you could thrash around evening time, or you probably won't rest by any means.
One investigation of 2,316 individuals uncovered that those experiencing a larger number of distressing episodes were at an essentially higher gamble of sleep deprivation. Restlessness can then prompt a large group of issues, including exhaustion, mindset swings, and absence of concentration.
However, rest isn't the main setback. Constant pressure has likewise been connected to

cerebrum shrinkage and cognitive decline. In one review, high cortisol levels were connected to more modest all-out cerebrum volumes, changes in the mind white matter, and unacceptable execution on a few memory and mental tasks. In another review, specialists took a gander at 1,225 people and found those with higher cortisol levels had a more troublesome time recollecting explicit occasions.

When would it be a good idea for me to see my primary care physician about my cortisol levels? If you experience side effects of Cushing's condition or adrenal deficiency, contact your medical care supplier.

Cortisol is a fundamental chemical that influences a few parts of your body. While there are a few things you can do to attempt to restrict your pressure, and hence deal with your cortisol levels, some of the time having unusually high or low degrees of cortisol is beyond your control.

In the event that you experience side effects of high or low cortisol levels, for example, weight gain or misfortune and high or low circulatory strain, separately, reaching your medical services provider is significant. They can run a few straightforward tests to check whether your adrenal organs or pituitary organs are liable for your symptoms.

Obviously, cortisol assumes an essential part in our body's science. Along these lines, constantly undeniable levels can influence various different significant capabilities. Also, it powers the psychological, close-to-home, and actual weariness that accompanies burnout.

Considering that, we want to address something many refer to as adrenal exhaustion.

Decrease Pressure and Forestall Burnout

The clearest method for forestalling burnout is to eliminate the stressor. To take off from the issue that is overburdening your framework.

Notwithstanding, can we just be real? The vast majority of us can't do that not immediately. The greater part of our pressure is attached to things we partner with long haul soundness: our positions, our wellbeing, our funds, our connections. We stress over these issues since clashes there undermine our security. So how would it be advisable for you to respond when you need to figure out your pressure?

In the first place, recognize that you're worried. That is, maybe, the main step.

Then, pinpoint the wellspring of your pressure. Then discuss it with somebody. Connect with companions or family. Or on the other, hand look for proficient assistance by counseling your overall doctor or a specialist.

What Cortisol Means for Emotional wellness

To make sense of what cortisol can mean for psychological wellness, we should return to the situation where the land experienced a bunch of hungry lions. Presently, nowadays, the vast majority aren't experiencing wild creatures consistently. Yet, while the conditions around us are not the same as an eland or our old progenitors, our cerebrums are as yet prepared to answer dangers. They have been adjusted to see current feelings of trepidation and tension like seeing an eager lion. In any case, today, the survival reaction is bound to come from circumstances like giving a show, hitting up a party, or even contemplating something that makes you restless.

Fight or Flight

Generally, fight or flight— also called intense pressure — is something to be thankful for. If you unexpectedly see a vehicle steering into your path and your body sets off a pressure reaction, you will want to answer rapidly and move far away. Furthermore, in any event, when the body responds this way to a harmless circumstance, such as playing tennis with a companion, it can in any case be gainful because it gets you equipped to perform at full limit.

Issues start when intense pressure is set off by cultural or mental stressors as opposed to actual stressors, as typical as covering your bills, sitting in rush hour gridlock, or any event, answering an email. Your body is ready to act, yet there's very little it can do to move away from the apparent danger.

Your pulse and circulatory strain are raised, and your body is in overdrive in planning, however, there's no unmistakable hunter to fight off, and you're left drained. While survival is enacted, your energy is all coordinated toward the danger, and numerous other physical processes that are unimportant right now are eased back or stopped.

Also, issues deteriorate when that intense pressure transforms into constant pressure. Survival is an interaction that is intended for armada: Subsequent to getting away or managing what is going on, the body should get back to its not unexpected state. Cortisol and other chemical levels, pulse, and pulse are undeniably expected to return to a resting state

and frameworks like processing that were not fundamental for endurance at the
time to return to work.

Chronic Pressure Conditions.

Constant pressure is the point at which your fight or flight reaction gets enacted again and again or stays on for a really long time. The mileage that persistent pressure puts on your body is connected with various mental and actual medical problems, including:

- Tension
- Sorrow
- Stomach related issues
- Migraines
- Heart issues
- Trouble dozing
- Putting on weight
- Issues with memory and focus

To a limited extent, the drawn-out high cortisol levels provoked by constant pressure are remembered to create these issues.

"We think that our brains and bodies weren't intended to have that arrangement of stress reaction, which incorporates cortisol, turned on so much of the time.

While the connection between cortisol and the improvement of emotional wellness issues isn't totally obvious, "any reasonable person would agree that constant pressure can make us powerless against the advancement of mental diseases.

Instructions to Oversee Pressure and Cortisol Levels.

1. Thoughtfully assess your timetable and balance between serious and fun activities.

Just know where your work-life plan falls on the curve.No one will roll out the improvement for you. On the off chance that you've been exhausted and pushed for quite a long time, there exists a hard open-door cost for taking on too much work.

Analysts have found that pressure and uneasiness can put you at a higher gamble of creating type 2 diabetes.1 Stress straightforwardly influences chemical levels, including insulin levels. Stress can likewise prompt undesirable propensities like drinking an excess of liquor, unfortunate food decisions, and not getting sufficient rest — all of which can add to weight gain. Being overweight, thus, likewise raises the gamble of creating type 2 diabetes. In 2018, the CDC and American Diabetes Affiliation (ADA) displayed more than 10% of the whole U.S. populace met models for some type of diabetes, with the rate quickly increasing. It can feel startling and overpowering to change occupations, professions, or areas. As somebody who by and by made a stupendous life shift to decrease feelings of anxiety, I can't pressure enough (seriously) how unimaginable I felt later. I lost 15 lbs and rested magnificently without precedent for 12 years, which carries me to my next idea.

2. Practice sound rest cleanliness.

Disturbed circadian rhythms and rest cycles add to unpredictable degrees of cortisol and development chemicals. This can cause glucose motions and weight gain. **This is the way to rehearse solid rest cleanliness:**

- Head to sleep and ascend concurrently every day.
- Polish off caffeine just in the first part of the day, and try not to eat or drink liquor 2 hours before bed. This invigorates the stomach-related framework when you ought to be slowing down for rest.
- Make a peaceful, dull, and cool spot for rest. The bed ought to just be utilized for rest and sex - don't work, stare at the television, or complete daytime errands in bed. It might sound senseless, yet this is a piece of molding the psyche into knowing that once you are sleeping, now is the ideal time to rest.
- Stay away from splendid screens 1-2 hours before bed, as this lets the psyche

know that the sun is out, which hinders
the mind's normal discharge of melatonin.
This chemical assists our minds with
entering the main phase of rest.

- Try not to enact content, for example,
web-based entertainment content and
news that may be setting off 1-2 hours
before bed.

3. Protect your brain and treat psychological wellness issues.

On the off chance that you experience the ill
effects of misery, nervousness, dietary problems,
or some other psychological well-being disease,
I urge you to look for treatment; which
incorporates seeing a medical care supplier and
beginning treatment. Living with persistent
pressure negatively affects the brain.

When discouraged, it can feel difficult to eat
well or exercise. Guiding can help as a type of
responsibility and assist you with making sound
limits throughout everyday life. For those with

dietary issues, many endeavors to lighten their pressure with profound eating. Try not to stall out in this endless loop.

There are various ways of pondering, and an ordinary practice can further develop your pressure reaction.

4. Practice careful reflection.

Yet again concentrates on showing that care reflection and acknowledgment practices lower pressure reactivity. Suggest doing this toward the beginning of the day and during the day. Track down a tranquil spot, sit serenely, and notice the brain for only 5 minutes; two times a day. Numerous fantastic webcasts and recordings online can direct you through contemplation rehearsals.

5. Attempt a ketogenic diet.

Current ketogenic rules suggest consuming the accompanying dissemination: 55-60% fat, 30-35% protein, and 5-10% carbs. Eating exceptionally handled food that is high in sugar adds to uneasiness, stress, and weight gain.

Since ketosis causes a crucial biochemical change in metabolic fuel for the cerebrum, ketosis brings about a profoundly loosening upstate, which can marginally improve feeling worried.

6. Work out

Broad exploration exhibits that normal activity really lessens feelings of anxiety. The practice has cardioprotective advantages, further develops rest quality, works with weight reduction, and numerous other medical advantages.

Rules suggest practicing for 30 mins 4-5 times each week. This can include:

strolling 1-2 miles around the area
Joining a rec center
Getting another game
Partaking in web-based practice recordings
In the event that you have joint issues or persistent agony, swimming is a great other option

Investing energy in nature and appreciating customary activity are great ways of making due stress.

Make a move to Lessen Pressure.

If you have any desire to completely change yourself then transform yourself. On the off chance that you need something you've never had, you should do
something you won't ever do.
I as of late scaled back my vocation and my work hours; it at first felt overpowering. I realize that constant high pressure causes a ton of damage to the body; more than expanding glucose levels.
The cost for many everyday items with persistent pressure ages the body — and it can take the brain with it.
While you're attempting to get in shape, it gets more troublesome with raised cortisol levels battling your eating and exercise endeavors. At

the point when you bring down your feelings of anxiety, you'll see an improvement in:

- Keeping up with stable glucose
- Weight reduction
- State of mind
- Nature of rest

I realize I saw these advantages, and I wouldn't exchange my well-being for all the cash in the world.

Chapter Four.

Do cortisol levels influence weight?

Among the various variables affecting your body weight, chemical guidelines are a significant one.
While chemicals, for example, cortisol are generally kept within a tight reach by your body's endocrine framework, there are sure circumstances in which they can turn out to be low or raised.

Significant levels might advance overeating.

Little ascents in cortisol levels in light of pressure are ordinary and not prone to cause negative secondary effects.

However, on specific occasions, cortisol levels might remain persistently raised.
This is generally because of stress or a condition like Cushing's disorder, which causes blood levels of cortisol to stay high.
At the point when cortisol levels stay raised, the accompanying after-effects might happen

- weight gain
- hypertension
- exhaustion
- changes in the state of mind
- touchiness
- flushed face
- diminishing skin
- trouble concentrating
- insulin obstruction

At the point when under constant pressure, it could be hard to keep up with energizing dietary patterns.

One concentrate in 59 sound ladies found a relationship between raised cortisol levels and an expansion in craving, which might actually advance weight gain

Furthermore, one more review found a relationship between a higher cortisol reaction and a higher measure of gut fat in a gathering of 172 people, recommending that higher cortisol might prompt overeating
All things considered, levels of pressure and cortisol aren't generally straightforwardly related, consequently, more information is expected to lay out an immediate relationship.

Low levels might cause weight reduction.

Similarly, as high cortisol levels might cause weight gain, low levels might cause weight reduction in certain occurrences.
The most outrageous model is Addison's sickness, a condition in which your body doesn't deliver sufficient cortisol.

The most outstanding side effects of low cortisol incorporates:

- diminished craving and weight reduction
- weakness
- low glucose
- salt desires
- unsteadiness
- queasiness, heaving, or stomach torment
- muscle or bone torment

While high cortisol levels might appear to be more normal, it's essential to know about the impacts of low cortisol also.

Persistently raised cortisol levels might advance gorging and weight gain, though low cortisol levels might prompt weight reduction on certain occasions.

The most effective method to forestall and battle weight gain because of cortisol levels.

While there might be numerous stressors in your day-to- day existence that possibly add to raised cortisol, there are a few powerful strategies for dealing with your levels and forestalling or battling weight gain.

1. Remain dynamic

One of the principal ways of combating weight gain is to participate in normal actual work. Normal activity has been related to a decrease in feelings of anxiety and permits you to be stronger when stressors introduce themselves In addition, practicing animates the arrival of endorphins, which are feel-great synthetic substances that advance bliss and can assist with overseeing pressure.

Normal actual work can likewise advance weight reduction or weight the executives because of the calories consumed while working out.

2. Practice careful eating

One more amazing asset for overseeing weight gain because of stress is rehearsing careful, or instinctive, eating.

Care comes from a Buddhist idea of significance to being completely present and mindful of what you're doing at a given second.

Careful eating applies this idea to food, empowering you to be completely mindful of your eating experience, including explicit signs, like yearning, completion, taste, and surface.

One enormous cross-sectional review found a relationship between the act of natural eating and lower body weight.

A basic method for beginning rehearsing carefully is to do with interruptions at dinners, permitting you to be completely mindful of craving and totality signals.

3. Speak to a specialist or dietitian

One more possible method for managing weight gain that could be connected with high cortisol levels is to talk with a certified expert, like a therapist or enrolled dietitian.

A specialist can help you in concocting a few methodologies to decrease general pressure, which thus might assist you with dealing with close-to-home eating.

Then again, a dietitian can furnish nourishment schooling to outfit you with the instruments you really want to settle on additional empowering choices encompassing food.

The double-prong way to deal with further develop your food propensities and profound prosperity is an amazing move toward forestalling or battling weight gain.

4. Get more rest

Rest is a usually neglected variable that essentially affects cortisol levels and potential weight gain.

Disturbances to your rest design — whether constant or intense — can advance an unfortunate expansion in cortisol levels.

Over the long haul, this can adversely affect your digestion and cause an expansion in specific chemicals connected with craving and hunger, possibly prompting weight gain. Hence, guaranteeing that you're getting satisfactory rest every night can go quite far toward keeping up with solid cortisol levels. The overall proposal for rest is 7-9 hours out each evening, however this shifts by age and different variables.

5. Practice reflection

One more expected apparatus for overseeing cortisol levels is contemplation.

The reason for contemplation is to prepare your psyche to concentrate and divert your considerations.

While a few sorts of contemplation exist, the most generally rehearsed ones are careful,

profound, centered, development, mantra, and supernatural.
Despite which you pick, rehearsing contemplation has been related to a decrease in cortisol levels in different populations.

Furthermore, contemplation might try and help work on the nature of your rest.

Chapter Five

Cortisol and infertility.

What Does Pressure Do to fertility?

One of the fundamental reasons pressure represses origination appears to have its foundations in a transformative system. As animal types, on the off chance that we were excessively worried, it implied it was anything but a protected opportunity to carry a baby into the world in view of starvation or absence of haven or assault from wild creatures. The issue is that now the stressors we are under are altogether different than they were 100, 500, or even a long time back however we actually answer pressure in the very same manner we did many quite a while back - we produce cortisol as a component of the 'flight or battle system' that sets us up to overcome, or take off from, risk.

Basically, when couples are desperate on their attempting to get pregnant can be one of the most distressing occasions for some couples and frequently, individuals don't understand exactly how much pressure they are under. Stress, whether intense or persistent, is a critical component with regard to fruitfulness and well-being. As a culture, we as a whole encounter different types of weight consistently; but it is our capacity to recuperate and mend from it that has an effect on the mileage on the adrenal organs and regenerative chemicals.

Stress and Fertility.

The explanation that stress can influence both male and female fruitfulness is established in our chemicals. Our sex chemicals (estrogen, progesterone for ladies, and testosterone for men) and our primary pressure chemical (cortisol) are totally produced using cholesterol. Cholesterol is, as a matter of fact, the foundation of all our steroid chemicals.

There are two fundamental sequences that these chemicals can take from the cholesterol atom. One produces testosterone and estrogen while the other produces progesterone and afterward cortisol. At the point when guys are anxious, the accentuation on chemical creation is shunted away from testosterone and towards making cortisol. At the point when females are anxious, their chemical creation is shunted from progesterone and towards cortisol. Basically, when men are focused on their testosterone drops and when ladies are focused on their progesterone drops.

For ideal fertility men need sound testosterone levels to create a lot of solid sperm - solid, direct swimmers with a decent morphology imperative for making the long excursion from the testicles to the female fallopian tube.

For ladies, progesterone levels are required basically for saving the uterine covering set up for a treated egg to embed into. Low degrees of progesterone leads to a short luteal stage which may not give sufficient time after ovulation for a treated egg to root into the uterine covering firmly. On the off chance that progesterone levels are not sufficiently high or they drop excessively fast then this will set off the uterine covering to shed causing the beginning of a feminine period. Low progesterone levels can likewise cause unsuccessful labor in the early piece of a pregnancy; it requires 10 weeks for a placenta to be ready and one of the many positions of the placenta is to create progesterone. This really intends that, until the 10th week, ladies are depending on the corpus luteum (or shell of the egg) in the ovary to deliver satisfactory measures of progesterone to keep up with the pregnancy. In the event that the lady has been under intense or ongoing pressure, her body focuses on cortisol creation over progesterone, and accordingly, her blood levels of progesterone drop.

Handling Pressure and Infertility - Dealing with the Adrenals.

Cortisol is delivered by the adrenals, little organs that live on top of the kidneys and produce a large number, of which cortisol is the overwhelming one. The adrenal organs assume a critical part in ripeness, but their job in the ordinary clinical model is neglected. The reality is this:

Supporting your adrenal glands supports your fertility.

Sadly, there are no convenient solutions for the adrenal organs. The condition of our adrenal organs is the amount of numerous long periods of stress, less than stellar eating routine and way of life and it might require numerous months to reestablish them to ideal wellbeing. In any case, that doesn't imply that making changes presently will not quickly affect your well-being and richness.

Advancing adrenal well-being, whether you have excessive or too little cortisol, is a similar methodology. The principal treatment contrast will be in the selection of botanicals and whether you really want support diminishing high cortisol.

Here are some top eating regimens and way-of-life tips to work on your adrenal well-being and your fruitfulness.

Diet

Diet assumes a significant part in advancing fruitfulness and most ladies who are attempting to consider are now wiping out caffeine and liquor and dealing with eating a better eating routine. Eating an eating routine that puts less "stress" on the adrenal organs decreases raised cortisol and keeps up with sound levels of the conceptive chemicals required for ripeness, for all kinds of people.

The principal chemical delivered by the adrenal organs is cortisol whose fundamental occupation is to manage blood glucose levels (our glucose). The point when our glucose levels drop too low is viewed as a "stressor" on the body making the mind trigger the adrenal organs to deliver more cortisol. Cortisol then attempts to amend what is going on by placing more glucose into the blood, essentially from stores in the liver. So one method for decreasing this additional development of cortisol is to keep away from that glucose plunge by eating 3 feasts (and conceivably 1 or 2 bites) each day, this will assist with controlling your glucose levels by staying away from emotional pinnacles and boxes. A sluggish consistent ascent and decline of blood glucose are less upsetting on the adrenal organs and the pancreas which produces insulin to carry the glucose from the blood and into the cell so attempt to keep away from dinners that are high in sugar and refined starches and that contain sound fat, fiber, and protein as this will give you a consistent ascent in glucose after a feast rather than a sharp spike.

Way of life

This is principally about the pressure on the executives. We as a whole have pressure yet it is learning procedures to manage that pressure that is critical. One of the most amazing ways of decreasing the abundance of cortisol is through exhalation. The yogis have it right when they say everything without a doubt revolves around the breath. Investing some peaceful energy alone consistently and zeroing in on sluggish consistent breaths can do wonders for disposing of an overabundance of cortisol. Furthermore, oxygen-consuming activity is additionally significant for diminishing cortisol. This is one reason we feel so good after working out. Certain individuals learn contemplation or study other unwinding procedures,

Bio-criticism. I prescribe attempting various methods to figure out which one is best for you.

Rest

Alluded to as great rest cleanliness, this implies attempting to get a normal of 8 hours of rest consistently with the initial 1-2 hours happening before 12 PM when cortisol levels begin to climb. In the event that you stay up past the point of no return, you will find it harder to nod off in view of cortisol's circadian mood. Cortisol levels ought to be at their most elevated in the first part of the day and least at night; on the off chance that we hit the sack more like 10 pm, we are following the ordinary hormonal musicality of the body and great rest cycles lessen the weight on the body.

Supplements

There are vitamins that are good for supporting the adrenal glands and balancing cortisol levels.
Vitamin C
Vitamin B Complex

Vitamin B5 as Pantethine
Vitamin B6 as Pyridoxine

Zinc

Progesterone
For some ladies, adding progesterone
supplementation after ovulation might be
essential. It is desirable over getting bio-
indistinguishable progesterone from an
intensified drug store

Chapter Six

The most effective method to gauge your cortisol levels.

What is a Cortisol Test?

A cortisol test estimates the degree of cortisol in your blood, pee, or spit to check whether your levels are normal. If your cortisol levels are excessively high or excessively low, it might mean you have an issue with your adrenal organs, an issue with your pituitary organ, or a growth that makes cortisol.

On account of pee tests, patients will for the most part have to gather their pee north of 24 hours. Then again, because hair develops all the more leisurely, how much cortisol in hair can be tried to perceive how much cortisol has been surrounding the body over a more stretched-out period — as long as a while. All the more as of late, researchers have been chipping away at creating wearable sensors that can screen cortisol levels.

Elevated degrees of cortisol may likewise occur on the off chance that you take enormous dosages of specific steroid drugs, like prednisone, for quite a while. What's more, low levels might occur assuming you stop the medication unexpectedly.

Without treatment, cortisol levels that are too high or too low can be intense.

Different names: urinary cortisol, salivary cortisol, free cortisol, blood cortisol, and plasma cortisol.

How Would You Test Your Cortisol Levels For Fertility?

Testing cortisol we can take a look at levels of testosterone (men) and progesterone levels (ladies). Both of these will be possible with a blood test. For guys, you need to test blood attracted in the morning for both free and add up to testosterone. For ladies you believe that should do a 'pooled progesterone test' - a solitary draw of progesterone won't give you enough information to be aware if your progesterone level is sufficiently high for fruitfulness purposes so you want to draw blood on 3 unique days beginning after ovulation. The amount of these 3 draws will give you precise progesterone esteem.

What is it utilized for?

a cortisol test is utilized to assist with diagnosing ailments that cause excessive or too little cortisol. These circumstances incorporate problems that influence the adrenal organs:

Cushing's condition is a problem that happens when your body has an excess of cortisol over a significant period.

Addison sickness is a condition wherein your adrenal organs are harmed and can't make sufficient cortisol.

Optional adrenal deficiency is a condition wherein your adrenal organs don't make sufficient cortisol because your pituitary organ isn't working as expected.

Cortisol testing is likewise used to screen treatment for these circumstances.

For what reason do I want a cortisol test?

You might require a cortisol test on the off chance that you have side effects of a condition that influences cortisol levels.

Side effects of Cushing's disorder (an excess of cortisol) may include:

- Barrenness
- Weight gain

- Slight arms and legs
- Round face
- Expanded fat around the foundation of the neck or between the shoulder bones
- Simple swelling
- Wide purple streaks on the stomach, bosoms, hips, and under the arms
- Muscle shortcoming

Normal side effects of Addison's sickness and the adrenal deficiency (insufficient cortisol) may incorporate

- Long-lasting fatigue
- Muscle shortcoming
- Deficiency of appetite
- Weight loss
- Abdominal (belly)pain.

End

Cortisol is a chemical that is mostly delivered on the occasion of pressure. Cortisol has numerous significant capabilities in the body. Having the right cortisol balance is fundamental for human well-being and you can have issues if you produce excessively or too little cortisol.
Cortisol is likewise required for the survival reaction, which is a solid, regular reaction to saw dangers. How much cortisol is created is exceptionally directed by your body to guarantee the equilibrium is right.
Cortisol as an expert chemical that influences the human body in various ways, fighting the impacts at the beginning phase provides the body with the suitable proportion of cortisol levels required in our body.